Timeless plate :

Anti aging tips for women.

By

Freda Shaw

Copyright

About the Author

Introducing Freda G. Shaw, a seasoned author weaving together her passion for plant science and the artistry of culinary creation. Armed with a degree in Plant Science, specializing in Botany, Freda explores the intricate world of plants, unveiling their nutritional richness and diverse flavors.

Freda's journey takes a captivating turn as she enters the realm of gastronomy with adept culinary skills. Her mastery transforms plant-based ingredients into timeless culinary treasures, infusing a delightful essence into the world of timeless plates.

In "Timeless Plate: A Culinary Journey through Plant-inspired Delights," Freda generously imparts her wealth of knowledge, guiding readers on a journey toward a balanced and sustainable approach to eating. The book authentically mirrors her expertise, inviting readers to savor the harmonious fusion of plant science and culinary excellence.

Introduction

Step into a world where each meal is a celebration of life and a key to unlocking the secrets of timeless living. "Timeless Plate: Unlock the Secrets of Youthful Living with Swift Anti-Aging Culinary Tips" invites you to embrace a culinary philosophy that goes beyond the ordinary – a philosophy that views the plate as a canvas for creating a vibrant and enduring life.

The Timeless Plate concept is rooted in the belief that what we choose to consume plays a pivotal role in our journey towards a youthful and energetic existence. It's not just about prolonging life; it's about savoring each moment with vitality, grace, and a plate filled with goodness. In these pages, we will explore the fascinating interplay between nutrition, age-defying ingredients, and the art of preparing meals that nourish both body and spirit.

As we navigate the realms of anti-aging cuisine, let the Timeless Plate be your guide, offering insights, recipes, and a renewed perspective on the profound connection between what you eat and how you live. Get ready to embark on a culinary adventure that transcends time itself. Welcome to the world of the Timeless Plate!

The impact of nutrition on aging

Aging, a natural and intricate process, unfolds gradually throughout the human lifespan. From the early stages of adulthood, a subtle symphony of changes marks the passage of time, impacting both mental and physical faculties. As this journey progresses, the impact of nutrition on aging becomes increasingly evident, offering a gateway to influence the pace and quality of this inevitable transformation.

Our choice of food emerges as a powerful determinant in shaping the aging trajectory. Essential nutrients found in a well-balanced diet act as catalysts, influencing cellular processes and contributing to the overall maintenance of bodily functions. The intricate dance between antioxidants and free radicals, fueled by the foods we consume, becomes a decisive factor in mitigating oxidative stress—a key player in the aging process.

Inflammation, a natural response that can turn detrimental with age, finds its balance on the plate. Opting for anti-inflammatory foods becomes a strategic move in managing the chronic inflammation associated with aging, contributing to the preservation of overall health.

Moreover, the interplay of sugars and proteins, known as glycation, introduces another layer to the aging narrative. Choosing foods with anti-glycation properties becomes a means of slowing down this process, potentially reducing the wear and tear on our cells over time.

In essence, our dietary choices become a form of intervention in the aging process. A nutrient-rich and thoughtfully curated plate can serve as a shield against the ravages of time, promoting cellular health and potentially slowing down the rate at which our bodies age. As we navigate the complex landscape of aging, let each bite be a conscious step towards nourishing not just our bodies but the timeless vitality that accompanies us on this profound journey.

The foundation of anti aging cuisine

At the heart of the quest for timeless living lies the foundation of anti-aging cuisine—a culinary philosophy that transcends mere sustenance to become a beacon for vitality and longevity. Rooted in the understanding that what we consume shapes the very fabric of our well-being, anti-aging cuisine serves as the architectural blueprint for a life marked by resilience and enduring health.

- Nutritional Alchemy:

The foundation of anti-aging cuisine is built upon the principles of nutritional alchemy, where each ingredient is chosen not just for flavor but for its transformative impact on cellular health. Essential nutrients become the alchemical elements, working synergistically to nourish and rejuvenate the body from within.

- Superfoods as Cornerstones:

Anti-aging cuisine embraces the concept of superfoods as cornerstones—ingredients rich in antioxidants, vitamins, and other bioactive compounds that go beyond basic nutrition. These culinary gems become the pillars of vitality, contributing to cellular repair and defense against the oxidative stress that accompanies aging.

- Balancing Act:

A key tenet of anti-aging cuisine is the delicate balance struck in crafting meals that are not only delicious but also nutritionally dense. It is a fusion of taste and health, where the plate becomes a canvas for creating a harmonious symphony of flavors and nutrients.

- Culinary Techniques for Preservation:

The foundation extends to culinary techniques that preserve the nutritional integrity of ingredients. Anti-aging cuisine explores cooking methods that retain essential vitamins and minerals, ensuring that the benefits of each bite are maximized for cellular health.

- Holistic Integration:

Beyond individual ingredients, anti-aging cuisine integrates a holistic approach to well-being. It recognizes the interconnectedness of lifestyle factors such as hydration, exercise, and stress management, weaving them seamlessly into the fabric of a lifestyle designed for longevity.

- Adaptability and Evolution:

Anti-aging cuisine is not a rigid doctrine but a dynamic and adaptable philosophy. It evolves with scientific insights, culinary innovations, and individual preferences. It encourages a mindful and informed approach to food choices, acknowledging that each person's journey towards timeless living is unique.

In essence, the foundation of anti-aging cuisine is a commitment to nourishing the body, mind, and spirit through the artful selection and preparation of food. It is a celebration of the profound connection between what we eat and how we age—a journey where the plate becomes a palette for crafting a life that stands the test of time.

Understanding aging at the cellular level

This unveils the intricate biological symphony that unfolds within our bodies over time. At the core of this exploration lies the recognition that aging is not a singular event but a nuanced and dynamic process involving a myriad of cellular changes. Delving into the cellular tapestry provides insights into the very essence of how our bodies evolve as the years pass.

- Telomeres and the Biological Clock:

One key element in understanding cellular aging is the role of telomeres. These protective caps at the end of our chromosomes act as a biological clock, gradually shortening with each cell division. As telomeres diminish, cells may undergo senescence, contributing to the overall aging of tissues and organs.

- DNA Maintenance and Repair:

Aging is intricately tied to the integrity of our DNA. Over time, exposure to environmental factors and internal processes can result in DNA damage. Cellular mechanisms for maintenance and repair become vital in preserving genetic information and preventing the accumulation of errors that can lead to aging-related issues.

- Mitochondria: Energy Centers and Aging Sentinels:

Mitochondria, the energy powerhouses of cells, play a dual role in aging. On one hand, they provide the energy needed for cellular functions; on the other, they are susceptible to damage and dysfunction over time. Mitochondrial health becomes a crucial aspect in understanding how cells age and impact overall vitality.

- Apoptosis: Programmed Cell Death and Renewal:

The controlled process of apoptosis, or programmed cell death, is a fundamental mechanism in cellular aging. It allows for the removal of damaged or unnecessary cells, contributing to tissue renewal. However, an imbalance in apoptosis can lead to issues such as tissue degeneration or excessive cell survival, both of which are associated with aging.

- Inflammation and Aging:

Chronic inflammation emerges as a key player in the cellular aging narrative. While acute inflammation is a necessary response to injury or infection, persistent low-grade inflammation can accelerate aging. Understanding the intricate interplay between inflammation and cellular function provides valuable insights into age-related health challenges.

Comprehending aging at the cellular level is akin to deciphering a complex language written within our very cells. It involves recognizing the delicate equilibrium between preservation and decline, renewal and senescence. As we navigate this microscopic landscape, we gain a deeper appreciation for the factors that influence the rate and quality of cellular aging—a knowledge that becomes foundational in the pursuit of strategies to promote healthy aging and vitality.

The role of nutrients in skin care health

The role of nutrients in skincare health is akin to providing the essential building blocks for a radiant and resilient complexion. As the body's largest organ, the skin relies on a diverse array of nutrients to maintain its structure, protect against environmental stressors, and promote overall well-being. Understanding the impact of specific nutrients on skin health unveils a holistic approach to nourishing and enhancing the skin's natural beauty.

- Vitamins as Skin Protectors:

Vitamin A: Known for its role in cell turnover, vitamin A aids in maintaining the skin's outer layer, promoting a smoother texture and reducing the appearance of fine lines.
Vitamin C: A powerful antioxidant, vitamin C helps protect the skin from oxidative stress, supports collagen synthesis for elasticity, and contributes to a brighter complexion.
Vitamin E: With its antioxidant properties, vitamin E helps defend the skin against free radicals, contributing to overall skin health and preventing premature aging.
Omega-3 Fatty Acids for Supple Skin:
Omega-3 fatty acids, found in fish oil and certain plant sources, play a crucial role in maintaining skin elasticity and hydration. These essential fats contribute to a healthy lipid barrier, preventing moisture loss and promoting a supple and youthful complexion.

- Antioxidants for Defense:

Various antioxidants, including vitamins mentioned earlier, as well as selenium and zinc, act as defenders against oxidative stress. By neutralizing free radicals, antioxidants help protect the skin from environmental damage, such as UV radiation and pollution, supporting a more resilient and youthful appearance.

- Collagen-Boosting Nutrients:

Collagen is a vital protein responsible for skin structure and elasticity. Nutrients like vitamin C, amino acids (proline and glycine), and copper contribute to collagen synthesis. Including these nutrients in the diet supports the skin's natural ability to maintain firmness and combat sagging.

- Hydration from Within:

While not a specific nutrient, adequate hydration is paramount for skin health. Water helps maintain skin moisture, preventing dryness and promoting a plump and vibrant complexion. Incorporating hydrating foods, such as fruits and vegetables with high water content, complements external skincare routines.

- Overall Diet and Skin Health:

A balanced and varied diet rich in fruits, vegetables, whole grains, and lean proteins provides a spectrum of nutrients essential for skin health. The synergy of these nutrients contributes to a comprehensive approach to skincare, fostering a radiant glow and supporting the body's natural defense mechanisms.

In essence, nourishing the skin from within through a nutrient-rich diet is a fundamental aspect of an effective skincare regimen. The combination of vitamins, essential fats, antioxidants, and collagen-boosting elements creates a foundation for healthy, resilient skin that radiates vitality.

Essential ingredients for youthful living

Essential ingredients for youthful living extend beyond mere sustenance, encompassing a spectrum of nutrients that support vitality, energy, and overall well-being. These elements, when incorporated into daily life, contribute to a holistic approach to youthful living, fostering physical resilience, mental acuity, and a vibrant spirit.

1. Antioxidant-Rich Foods:

A diet rich in antioxidants serves as a cornerstone for youthful living. Fruits and vegetables such as berries, leafy greens, and citrus fruits provide a diverse array of antioxidants that combat oxidative stress, promoting cell health and potentially slowing down the aging process.

2. Omega-3 Fatty Acids:
Found in fatty fish, flaxseeds, and walnuts, omega-3 fatty acids are essential for brain health, cardiovascular function, and maintaining supple skin. These healthy fats contribute to overall well-being and are integral to a youthful and resilient body.

3. Superfoods with Nutrient Density:
Incorporating nutrient-dense superfoods, such as chia seeds, kale, and spirulina, ensures a concentrated supply of vitamins, minerals, and phytonutrients. These powerhouse ingredients support optimal functioning of various bodily systems, promoting vitality and longevity.

4. Lean Proteins:
Proteins are fundamental for muscle maintenance, immune function, and overall energy levels. Lean protein sources like poultry, fish, tofu, and legumes provide essential amino acids necessary for bodily repair and rejuvenation.

5. Colorful Fruits and Vegetables:
The vibrant hues of fruits and vegetables signal a rich assortment of vitamins and minerals. A colorful plate not only pleases the palate but also delivers a broad spectrum of nutrients that contribute to skin health, immune function, and overall vitality.

6. Hydration:
Water is an indispensable ingredient for youthful living. Staying adequately hydrated supports skin hydration, aids digestion, and helps maintain overall bodily functions. Infusing hydration with herbal teas and hydrating foods enhances the overall approach to staying youthful.

7. Whole Grains for Sustained Energy:
Incorporating whole grains like quinoa, brown rice, and oats provides complex carbohydrates that release energy gradually, promoting sustained vitality throughout the day. These grains also contribute fiber for digestive health.

8. Probiotics for Gut Health:
A flourishing gut microbiome is linked to overall health, including immune function and mental well-being. Fermented foods like yogurt, kefir, and kimchi introduce beneficial probiotics that support a balanced and resilient gut.

9. Adequate Sleep:
While not a food ingredient, prioritizing adequate and quality sleep is a fundamental aspect of youthful living. During sleep, the body undergoes essential repair processes, contributing to physical and mental rejuvenation.

10. Mindful Practices:
Incorporating mindfulness practices, such as meditation and stress management techniques, serves as a non-negotiable ingredient for youthful living. These practices support mental resilience, emotional well-being, and overall life satisfaction.

By cultivating a lifestyle rich in these essential ingredients, individuals can create a robust foundation for youthful living, fostering a harmonious balance between physical health, mental vitality, and a zest for life.

Antioxidant rich foods

Antioxidant-rich foods are like superheroes for your health. They help protect your body from something called oxidative stress, which can damage your cells and contribute to aging and diseases. Including these foods in your diet can be a tasty way to boost your overall well-being.

- Berries:

Blueberries, strawberries, raspberries, and blackberries are packed with antioxidants. They not only taste delicious but also provide a burst of health-boosting compounds.

- Dark Leafy Greens:

Spinach, kale, and Swiss chard are loaded with antioxidants like vitamin C, vitamin E, and beta-carotene. These leafy greens are not only good for your skin but also support your overall health.

- Citrus Fruits:

Oranges, lemons, grapefruits, and limes are rich in vitamin C, a powerful antioxidant that helps your immune system and promotes healthy skin.

- Nuts and Seeds:

Almonds, walnuts, chia seeds, and flaxseeds are excellent sources of antioxidants. They also provide healthy fats, fiber, and other essential nutrients.

- Colorful Vegetables:

Bell peppers, tomatoes, carrots, and sweet potatoes get their vibrant colors from antioxidants. Including a variety of colorful veggies ensures a mix of beneficial compounds.

- Green Tea:

Green tea is not just a soothing beverage; it's also loaded with antioxidants called catechins. These compounds may contribute to heart health and overall well-being.

- Dark Chocolate:

Indulging in dark chocolate (in moderation) provides antioxidants called flavonoids. Look for chocolate with higher cocoa content for more health benefits.

- Red Grapes:

Red grapes contain resveratrol, an antioxidant that has been linked to various health benefits, including heart health.

- Turmeric:

This spice contains curcumin, a potent antioxidant with anti-inflammatory properties. Adding turmeric to your meals can be a flavorful way to boost your antioxidant intake.

- Broccoli:

Broccoli is a nutritional powerhouse with antioxidants like sulforaphane. It's not only good for your overall health but also supports a healthy immune system.

Including a variety of antioxidant-rich foods in your diet is like giving your body a shield against free radicals. These foods not only taste good but also contribute to your overall health and well-being.

omega -3 fatty acids and their benefits

Omega-3 fatty acids are like special helpers for your body, offering a range of benefits that support your health. These healthy fats are essential, meaning your body needs them but can't produce them on its own. Including omega-3-rich foods in your diet can contribute to a happy and healthy you.

1. Heart Health:

Omega-3s are heart-friendly! They can help lower bad cholesterol levels, reduce triglycerides, and support overall heart health. Eating fish like salmon, mackerel, and sardines is a tasty way to get these benefits.

2. Brain Boost:

Your brain loves omega-3s! They play a crucial role in brain development and function. Including fatty fish, walnuts, and flaxseeds in your diet may help improve memory and cognitive function.

3. Joint Health:

Omega-3s can be like a friend to your joints. They may help reduce inflammation, easing stiffness and discomfort. Fish oil supplements or incorporating fish into your meals can be beneficial.

4. Good Mood and Mental Health:

These special fats are linked to better mood and mental well-being. Including omega-3-rich foods may be helpful in managing stress, anxiety, and even depression.

5. Eye Health:

Omega-3s are like superheroes for your eyes! They are an essential component of the retina, contributing to good eyesight. Fish, particularly fatty fish, is great for promoting eye health.

6. Skin Benefits:

Omega-3s can be your skin's best friend. They help maintain skin health, keeping it moisturized and potentially reducing signs of aging. Include fish, chia seeds, and flaxseeds for a skin-loving boost.

7. Pregnancy and Early Development:

For moms-to-be, omega-3s are crucial for the development of the baby's brain and eyes. Eating fish or taking omega-3 supplements during pregnancy can contribute to a healthy start for your little one.

8. Anti-Inflammatory Properties:

Omega-3s have anti-inflammatory powers, helping your body fight inflammation. This can be beneficial for conditions like arthritis and other inflammatory disorders.

9. Immune System Support:

Including omega-3s in your diet can give your immune system a boost. They may help your body respond better to infections and support overall immune function.

10. Weight Management:
- Omega-3s might be helpful in weight management by supporting healthy metabolism. Including fish and other omega-3 sources in a balanced diet can be part of a weight-conscious lifestyle.

Remember, it's essential to get omega-3s from your diet because your body can't make them. Including a variety of foods like fatty fish, nuts, seeds, and plant oils ensures you're reaping the benefits of these fantastic fats for your overall well-being.

Super foods for anti aging

Superfoods for anti-aging are like a gift from nature, packed with nutrients that can help keep you looking and feeling youthful. Including these powerful foods in your diet can be a delicious way to support your skin, boost energy, and promote overall well-being.

1. Berries:

Blueberries, strawberries, and raspberries are rich in antioxidants, helping fight free radicals and potentially slowing down the aging process. They're like little nutrient powerhouses for your skin.

2. Avocado:

Avocados are a superfood for smooth and radiant skin. Packed with healthy fats and vitamins, they support skin hydration and may reduce the appearance of wrinkles.

3. Leafy Greens:

Spinach, kale, and Swiss chard are anti-aging champions. Loaded with vitamins, minerals, and antioxidants, they contribute to skin health, boost collagen production, and support overall vitality.

4. Fatty Fish:

Salmon, mackerel, and sardines are rich in omega-3 fatty acids. These healthy fats support skin elasticity, reduce inflammation, and promote a youthful glow.

5. Nuts and Seeds:

Almonds, walnuts, chia seeds, and flaxseeds are like tiny anti-aging packages. Packed with antioxidants, healthy fats, and essential nutrients, they support skin, heart, and brain health.

6. Dark Chocolate:

Dark chocolate (in moderation) is a delicious treat with anti-aging benefits. It contains antioxidants that can help protect your skin from damage and promote overall well-being.

7. Green Tea:

Green tea is a sip of youth! Rich in antioxidants, particularly catechins, it may help protect your skin from sun damage and support a radiant complexion.

8. Turmeric:

Turmeric is like a golden secret for anti-aging. It contains curcumin, known for its anti-inflammatory and antioxidant properties, which may support overall skin health.

9. Tomatoes:

Tomatoes are not just tasty; they're also packed with antioxidants, including lycopene. Lycopene helps protect your skin from sun damage and promotes a healthy, youthful appearance.

10. Greek Yogurt:
- Greek yogurt is a superfood for your gut and skin. It's rich in probiotics, which support a healthy digestive system, and its protein content contributes to skin firmness.

11. Broccoli:
- Broccoli is an anti-aging powerhouse. Packed with vitamins, minerals, and antioxidants, it supports collagen production and helps combat the signs of aging.

12. Watermelon:
- Watermelon is not just refreshing; it's great for your skin. Rich in hydration and antioxidants like lycopene, it contributes to skin health and a youthful glow.

Incorporating these superfoods into your diet provides a tasty and nutritious way to support your anti-aging journey. Remember, it's the combination of a balanced diet, hydration, and a healthy lifestyle that contributes to looking and feeling your best over time.

Culinary techniques for timeless cooking

Culinary techniques for timeless cooking embrace the art of preparing meals in a way that not only delights the taste buds but also supports long-lasting health and well-being. These techniques focus on preserving nutrients, enhancing flavors, and creating a balance that stands the test of time.

1. Steaming:

Steaming is a gentle cooking method that helps retain the natural goodness of foods. It preserves vitamins and minerals while keeping the flavors intact. This technique is ideal for vegetables, fish, and even grains.

2. Grilling:

Grilling adds a smoky flavor to foods while allowing excess fats to drip away. It's a timeless technique that imparts a delicious taste to meats and vegetables, making meals both flavorful and healthy.

3. Roasting:

Roasting involves cooking food in an oven at a high temperature. This method caramelizes sugars in vegetables, intensifies flavors, and gives a golden, crispy texture to meats. It's a versatile and enduring technique.

4. Slow Cooking:

Slow cooking allows flavors to meld together over time. It's a method that transforms tough cuts of meat into tender delights and creates rich, hearty stews. The slow infusion of flavors makes dishes timeless and comforting.

5. Fermentation:

Fermentation is a traditional technique that not only preserves foods but also enhances their nutritional profile. Foods like kimchi, sauerkraut, and yogurt made through fermentation introduce beneficial probiotics for gut health.

6. Sous Vide:

Sous vide, a method of cooking food in vacuum-sealed bags at precise temperatures, ensures even cooking and retention of nutrients. This modern technique combines precision with the timeless goal of preserving the essence of ingredients.

7. Raw Preparation:

Embracing raw food preparation, such as salads and carpaccios, allows you to savor the natural flavors and nutrients of fresh ingredients. It's a timeless way to enjoy the vibrant essence of fruits and vegetables.

8. Herbs and Spices:

Using herbs and spices generously adds depth and complexity to dishes without relying on excessive salt or unhealthy fats. This culinary technique allows you to create enduring flavors while supporting overall health.

9. Simmering and Braising:

Simmering and braising involve cooking food slowly in liquid. These techniques transform tougher cuts of meat into tender creations and infuse dishes with rich, complex flavors over time.

10. Mindful Pairing:
- Timeless cooking involves mindful pairing of ingredients. Combining complementary flavors, textures, and colors creates a harmonious dish that transcends trends, ensuring a timeless appeal.

11. Minimal Processing:
- Keeping food processing to a minimum helps preserve the inherent qualities of ingredients. Minimal processing retains nutrients and allows the true flavors to shine through, contributing to the timeless nature of a dish.

By incorporating these culinary techniques into your cooking repertoire, you not only create delicious and enduring meals but also contribute to the nourishment and enjoyment of those who partake in the timeless experience of sharing a well-prepared dish.

healthy cooking methods

Healthy cooking methods are the foundation of creating nutritious and delicious meals. By choosing methods that preserve nutrients and minimize added fats, you can promote overall well-being without sacrificing flavor. Here are some healthy cooking techniques to consider:

1. Steaming:

Steaming involves cooking food over boiling water. It's a gentle method that retains nutrients, color, and flavor. Perfect for vegetables, fish, and even grains.

2. Grilling:

Grilling imparts a smoky flavor without excessive fats. Opt for lean proteins like chicken or fish and include colorful vegetables for a healthy and flavorful meal.

3. Baking and Roasting:

Baking and roasting use dry heat to cook food in the oven. This technique enhances flavors, caramelizes natural sugars, and requires minimal added fats. Great for vegetables, poultry, and whole grains.

4. Sautéing:

Sautéing involves cooking food quickly in a small amount of oil. Use heart-healthy oils like olive or avocado oil and incorporate a variety of colorful vegetables for added nutrients.

5. Broiling:

Broiling cooks food under high, direct heat. It's a quick method that adds a nice sear while allowing fats to drip away. Perfect for lean cuts of meat and fish.

6. Poaching:

Poaching involves gently simmering food in liquid. This low-fat method is excellent for delicate proteins like fish or eggs, preserving their tenderness and nutritional value.

7. Steaming in Packets (En Papillote):

Cooking in parchment paper or foil packets helps seal in flavors and nutrients. This method is versatile and allows for creative combinations of proteins and vegetables.

8. Boiling:

Boiling is a simple method that works well for vegetables, grains, and pasta. Be mindful of cooking times to prevent nutrient loss, and use the least amount of water necessary.

9. Stir-Frying:

Stir-frying quickly cooks small, uniform-sized pieces of food in a small amount of oil. Use vibrant vegetables and lean proteins for a nutrient-packed, colorful dish.

10. Raw or Minimal Cooking:
- Incorporating raw elements into your meals, such as salads or carpaccios, ensures you benefit from the full array of nutrients found in fresh produce.

11. Slow Cooking:
- Slow cooking is a hands-free method that transforms tough cuts of meat and infuses flavors over time. It's great for soups, stews, and hearty dishes.

12. Griddling:
- Griddling involves cooking on a flat surface with minimal oil. It's suitable for a variety of foods, including lean proteins and vegetables, providing a healthy and convenient cooking option.

13. Microwave Cooking:
- While not suitable for all foods, microwaving can be a quick and healthy cooking method for vegetables, grains, and proteins, helping to preserve nutrients.

By incorporating these healthy cooking techniques into your culinary routine, you can create meals that are not only tasty but also contribute to your overall health and well-being. Remember to focus on whole, fresh ingredients and minimize the use of unhealthy fats and excessive salt for optimal results.

Flavourful and nutrient preserving recipes

1. Steamed Salmon with Lemon and Herbs:
Healthy and full of Omega-3 fatty acids.

Ingredients:

4 salmon filets
1 lemon, sliced
Fresh herbs (such as dill, parsley, or thyme)
Salt and pepper to taste
Instructions:

Season the salmon filets with salt and pepper.
Place a few slices of lemon and a sprig of herbs on each filet.
Arrange the filets in a steamer basket over boiling water.
Cover and steam for 8-10 minutes or until the salmon is cooked through.
Serve with additional lemon wedges and a sprinkle of fresh herbs.

2. Roasted Vegetable Quinoa Bowl:
Packed with nutrients and flavor.

Ingredients:

1 cup quinoa, rinsed
2 cups mixed vegetables (e.g., bell peppers, zucchini, cherry tomatoes)
2 tablespoons olive oil
1 teaspoon dried herbs (such as oregano or thyme)
Salt and pepper to taste
Optional toppings: feta cheese, avocado, or a drizzle of balsamic glaze
Instructions:

Preheat the oven to 400°F (200°C).
Toss the mixed vegetables with olive oil, dried herbs, salt, and pepper.
Spread the vegetables on a baking sheet in a single layer.

Roast in the oven for 20-25 minutes or until the vegetables are tender and slightly caramelized.
While the vegetables are roasting, cook quinoa according to package instructions.
Assemble bowls with a base of quinoa and top with the roasted vegetables.
Add optional toppings like feta cheese, avocado slices, or a drizzle of balsamic glaze.

3. Lemon Garlic Herb Chicken Skewers:
Perfect for a light and protein-packed meal.

Ingredients:

1 lb boneless, skinless chicken breast, cut into cubes
Zest and juice of 1 lemon
3 cloves garlic, minced
Fresh herbs (rosemary, thyme, or oregano), chopped
Salt and pepper to taste
Cherry tomatoes and bell peppers for skewering
Instructions:

In a bowl, mix lemon zest, lemon juice, minced garlic, chopped herbs, salt, and pepper.
Marinate chicken cubes in the mixture for at least 30 minutes.
Thread marinated chicken, cherry tomatoes, and bell peppers onto skewers.
Grill or broil the skewers until the chicken is fully cooked and has a golden color.
Serve with a side of quinoa or a green salad.

4. Vegetarian Stir-Fry with Tofu:
A quick and nutrient-packed stir-fry.

Ingredients:

1 block firm tofu, pressed and cubed
Assorted vegetables (broccoli, bell peppers, snap peas, carrots)
2 tablespoons soy sauce
1 tablespoon sesame oil
1 tablespoon ginger, minced
2 cloves garlic, minced
Brown rice or quinoa for serving
Instructions:

In a wok or skillet, heat sesame oil and sauté ginger and garlic.
Add cubed tofu and stir-fry until golden.
Add assorted vegetables and continue to stir-fry until they are tender-crisp.
Pour in soy sauce and toss everything together until well-coated.
Serve over cooked brown rice or quinoa.

5. Mango Avocado Salsa Salmon:
Refreshing and rich in Omega-3s.

Ingredients:

4 salmon filets
1 ripe mango, diced
1 avocado, diced
1/4 cup red onion, finely chopped
Fresh cilantro, chopped
Juice of 1 lime
Salt and pepper to taste
Instructions:

Season salmon filets with salt and pepper and grill or bake until done.
In a bowl, combine diced mango, avocado, red onion, cilantro, and lime juice.
Spoon the mango avocado salsa over the grilled salmon.
Garnish with extra cilantro and serve with a side of quinoa or wild rice.

6. Mediterranean Chickpea Salad:
A refreshing salad with Mediterranean flavors.

Ingredients:

2 cans chickpeas, drained and rinsed
Cherry tomatoes, halved
Cucumber, diced
Kalamata olives, sliced
Feta cheese, crumbled
Red onion, finely chopped
Olive oil, lemon juice, and dried oregano for dressing
Instructions:

In a large bowl, combine chickpeas, cherry tomatoes, cucumber, olives, feta, and red onion.
In a small bowl, whisk together olive oil, lemon juice, and dried oregano for the dressing.
Pour the dressing over the salad and toss to coat.
Serve chilled as a light and nutritious meal or side dish.

7. Quinoa Stuffed Bell Peppers:
A wholesome and colorful dish.

Ingredients:

Bell peppers, halved and seeds removed

1 cup quinoa, cooked
Black beans, drained and rinsed
Corn kernels
Diced tomatoes
Taco seasoning or cumin, paprika, and chili powder
Shredded cheese (optional)
Instructions:

Preheat the oven to 375°F (190°C).
In a bowl, mix cooked quinoa, black beans, corn, diced tomatoes, and taco seasoning.
Stuff each bell pepper half with the quinoa mixture.
Top with shredded cheese if desired.
Bake for 20-25 minutes or until the peppers are tender.
Garnish with fresh cilantro and serve with salsa or Greek yogurt.

8. Herb-Crusted Baked Cod:
A light and flavorful fish dish.

Ingredients:

4 cod filets
Fresh herbs (such as parsley, dill, and chives), finely chopped
Lemon zest
Whole-grain mustard
Olive oil
Salt and pepper to taste
Instructions:

Preheat the oven to 400°F (200°C).
In a bowl, mix chopped herbs, lemon zest, mustard, olive oil, salt, and pepper.
Coat the cod filets with the herb mixture.
Place the filets on a baking sheet and bake for 15-20 minutes or until the fish flakes easily.
Serve with a side of steamed vegetables or quinoa.

9. Sweet Potato and Chickpea Curry:
A nourishing and aromatic curry.

Ingredients:

2 sweet potatoes, peeled and diced
1 can chickpeas, drained and rinsed
Coconut milk
Curry powder, turmeric, and cumin
Garlic and ginger, minced

Spinach leaves
Brown rice for serving
Instructions:

In a large pot, sauté garlic and ginger until fragrant.
Add diced sweet potatoes, chickpeas, and spices. Stir to coat.
Pour in coconut milk and simmer until sweet potatoes are tender.
Add spinach and cook until wilted.
Serve the curry over brown rice.

10. Caprese Quinoa Salad:
A refreshing and protein-packed salad.

Ingredients:

1 cup quinoa, cooked
Cherry tomatoes, halved
Fresh mozzarella balls, diced
Fresh basil leaves, torn
Balsamic glaze
Olive oil
Salt and pepper to taste
Instructions:

In a bowl, combine cooked quinoa, cherry tomatoes, mozzarella, and basil.
Drizzle with olive oil and balsamic glaze.
Season with salt and pepper to taste.
Toss gently to combine.
Serve as a light and satisfying salad.

These recipes incorporate a variety of flavors and nutrient-rich ingredients while preserving their goodness through thoughtful cooking methods. Enjoy these wholesome meals as part of a balanced and nutritious diet.

Creating balanced and anti aging meal

Creating a balanced and anti-aging meal involves combining nutrient-dense foods that promote overall well-being and support your body's natural defenses against aging. Here's a guide to crafting such a meal:

1. Lean Protein:
Include sources like fish, poultry, tofu, or legumes. Protein aids in muscle maintenance, supports immune function, and provides a feeling of fullness.
2. Colorful Vegetables:
Opt for a variety of colorful vegetables rich in antioxidants. Bell peppers, leafy greens, carrots, and tomatoes contribute vitamins, minerals, and phytonutrients that combat oxidative stress.
3. Healthy Fats:
Incorporate sources of healthy fats like avocados, nuts, seeds, and olive oil. These fats support skin health, help absorb fat-soluble vitamins, and contribute to overall well-being.
4. Whole Grains:
Choose whole grains such as quinoa, brown rice, or oats. They provide complex carbohydrates for sustained energy, fiber for digestion, and various essential nutrients.
5. Berries and Fruits:
Berries, rich in antioxidants, and fruits like apples and citrus add natural sweetness and provide essential vitamins. They contribute to skin health and overall vitality.
6. Probiotic-Rich Foods:
Include yogurt, kefir, or fermented vegetables for a dose of probiotics. These support gut health, influencing overall well-being and potentially impacting the aging process.
7. Herbs and Spices:
Flavor your meals with herbs and spices like turmeric, ginger, and garlic. They offer anti-inflammatory properties and add depth to the dish without relying on excess salt.
8. Omega-3 Fatty Acids:
Incorporate fatty fish like salmon or chia seeds and flaxseeds for plant-based omega-3s. These healthy fats support heart health, brain function, and may contribute to a youthful appearance.
9. Hydration:
Drink plenty of water throughout the day. Staying hydrated supports skin elasticity, aids digestion, and is essential for overall bodily functions.
10. Green Tea:
-Enjoy a cup of green tea. Rich in antioxidants, it may contribute to skin health and overall well-being.
11. Moderation and Mindful Eating:
 Practice portion control and mindful eating. Listen to your body's hunger and fullness cues, savoring each bite.
12. Limit Processed Foods:
 Minimize processed foods and refined sugars. Opt for whole, unprocessed foods to maximize nutrient intake and minimize potential sources of inflammation.

13. Include Anti-Aging Nutrients:
Ensure your meal includes nutrients like vitamin C, vitamin E, selenium, and beta-carotene, known for their anti-aging properties.

By incorporating these elements into your meals, you create a balanced and anti-aging dining experience. Emphasizing a variety of nutrient-rich foods not only supports your body's health but also contributes to a vibrant and youthful lifestyle.

Building nutrient rich plates

Building nutrient-rich plates involves incorporating a variety of foods that provide essential vitamins, minerals, antioxidants, and other beneficial compounds. Here's a guide to help you create plates that are not only delicious but also packed with nutritional value:

1. Colorful Vegetables:
Fill half your plate with a variety of colorful vegetables. Aim for a mix of leafy greens, peppers, tomatoes, carrots, and cruciferous veggies like broccoli and cauliflower. The vibrant colors indicate different nutrients and antioxidants.
2. Lean Protein:
Include a lean protein source to support muscle health and overall satiety. Options include grilled chicken, fish, tofu, legumes, or lean cuts of meat. Adjust portion sizes based on your dietary needs.
3. Whole Grains:
Choose whole grains to provide complex carbohydrates, fiber, and various nutrients. Options include quinoa, brown rice, whole wheat pasta, or farro. These grains contribute to sustained energy levels.
4. Healthy Fats:
Add sources of healthy fats for heart health and satiety. Avocado slices, nuts, seeds, or a drizzle of olive oil are excellent choices. Be mindful of portion sizes to manage calorie intake.
5. Fruits:
Include a serving of fresh fruits for natural sweetness and additional vitamins. Berries, apples, or citrus fruits are rich in antioxidants and add a refreshing touch.
6. Dairy or Dairy Alternatives:
Incorporate dairy or fortified dairy alternatives for calcium and vitamin D. Greek yogurt, low-fat milk, or fortified plant-based alternatives like almond or soy milk are good choices.
7. Herbs and Spices:
Flavor your dishes with herbs and spices instead of excessive salt. Fresh herbs like basil, cilantro, or mint, along with spices such as turmeric, cumin, and garlic, enhance taste without added sodium.
8. Probiotic Foods:

Include foods rich in probiotics for gut health. Yogurt with live cultures, kefir, sauerkraut, or kimchi are excellent choices to support your digestive system.
9. Hydration:
Don't forget to hydrate! Water is essential for overall health. Consider herbal teas or infused water with slices of cucumber, citrus, or berries for added flavor.
10. Mindful Portions:
- Pay attention to portion sizes to maintain a balanced intake of nutrients. Use smaller plates to help with portion control.
11. Variety and Seasonality:
- Embrace variety and seasonality. Include a diverse range of foods to ensure a broad spectrum of nutrients throughout the year.
12. Limit Processed Foods:
- Minimize processed and refined foods. Focus on whole, minimally processed options to maximize nutritional benefits.

By combining these elements, you create plates that are not only visually appealing but also provide a rich array of nutrients essential for overall health and well-being. Adjust portion sizes based on your individual needs and preferences, and enjoy the nourishing experience of nutrient-rich meals.

Meal planning for longevity

Meal planning for longevity involves making thoughtful choices to support overall health and well-being. By incorporating nutrient-dense foods, balanced meals, and mindful eating habits, you can create a meal plan that promotes longevity. Here's a guide to help you get started:

1. Plant-Centric Approach:
Prioritize plant-based foods such as fruits, vegetables, whole grains, legumes, nuts, and seeds. These foods are rich in antioxidants, fiber, and various micronutrients linked to longevity.
2. Variety of Colors:
Aim for a colorful plate by including a variety of fruits and vegetables. Different colors often signify distinct nutrients and antioxidants, providing a broad range of health benefits.
3. Lean Proteins:
Include lean protein sources like fish, poultry, tofu, legumes, and low-fat dairy. Protein is essential for muscle maintenance and overall bodily function.

4. Healthy Fats:

Choose sources of healthy fats, such as avocados, nuts, seeds, and olive oil. These fats contribute to heart health and provide satiety.
5. Whole Grains:

Opt for whole grains like quinoa, brown rice, oats, and whole wheat bread. Whole grains offer complex carbohydrates, fiber, and various nutrients.

6. Limit Processed Foods:

Minimize processed and refined foods, which often contain added sugars, unhealthy fats, and preservatives. Focus on whole, minimally processed options.

7. Mindful Portions:

Practice portion control to avoid overeating. Listen to your body's hunger and fullness cues, and savor each bite.

8. Hydration:

Stay well-hydrated by drinking plenty of water throughout the day. Proper hydration supports various bodily functions and overall health.

9. Include Antioxidant-Rich Foods:

Incorporate foods rich in antioxidants, such as berries, leafy greens, and colorful vegetables. Antioxidants help combat oxidative stress and inflammation.

10. Probiotic Foods:

- Support gut health by including probiotic-rich foods like yogurt, kefir, sauerkraut, or kimchi. A healthy gut is linked to overall well-being.

11. Herbs and Spices:

- Flavor your meals with herbs and spices instead of excessive salt. Herbs like rosemary, turmeric, and garlic have been associated with health benefits.

12. Intermittent Fasting:

- Consider incorporating intermittent fasting, a pattern of eating that alternates between periods of eating and fasting. Some studies suggest potential benefits for longevity.

13. Social and Enjoyable Meals:

- Share meals with friends and family. Social connections and the enjoyment of meals are linked to emotional well-being, which contributes to a longer, healthier life.

14. Seasonal and Local Foods:

- Choose seasonal and locally sourced foods when possible. They are often fresher and may retain more nutrients.

15. Stay Active:

- Complement your meal plan with regular physical activity. Exercise is a key component of a healthy lifestyle and longevity.

By incorporating these principles into your meal planning, you can create a balanced and nutritious approach that aligns with the goal of promoting longevity and overall well-being. Remember that individual needs may vary, so it's advisable to consult with a healthcare professional or a registered dietitian for personalized guidance.

lifestyle habit for youthful vitality

Adopting lifestyle habits that promote youthful vitality involves incorporating practices that support physical, mental, and emotional well-being. Here's a guide to cultivating habits that contribute to a vibrant and energized lifestyle:

1. Regular Exercise:
Engage in regular physical activity, including a mix of cardiovascular exercises, strength training, and flexibility exercises. Exercise promotes circulation, maintains muscle mass, and supports overall vitality.
2. Adequate Sleep:
Prioritize quality sleep by establishing a consistent sleep schedule. Aim for 7-9 hours of restful sleep each night to allow your body to rejuvenate and promote optimal cognitive function.
3. Balanced Nutrition:
Maintain a balanced and nutrient-rich diet with a variety of fruits, vegetables, lean proteins, whole grains, and healthy fats. Proper nutrition supports energy levels, skin health, and overall vitality.
4. Hydration:
Stay well-hydrated by drinking an ample amount of water throughout the day. Hydration is crucial for bodily functions, skin health, and maintaining energy levels.
5. Stress Management:
Practice stress-reducing techniques such as mindfulness, meditation, or deep breathing exercises. Chronic stress can accelerate aging, so finding effective ways to manage stress is essential for youthful vitality.

6. Sun Protection:
Protect your skin from sun damage by using sunscreen and adopting sun-safe practices. Sun protection helps prevent premature aging and maintains skin health.

7. Social Connections:
Cultivate and maintain strong social connections. Positive relationships and a supportive social network contribute to emotional well-being and a sense of youthful vitality.

8. Continual Learning:
Stimulate your mind through continual learning and engagement. Pursue hobbies, read, or engage in activities that challenge and inspire you, promoting cognitive vitality.

9. Mindful Eating:
Practice mindful eating by savoring each bite and paying attention to hunger and fullness cues. Mindful eating encourages a healthier relationship with food and supports overall well-being.

10. Limit Toxins:
- Minimize exposure to toxins by choosing natural cleaning products, avoiding excessive alcohol and tobacco use, and opting for organic foods when possible. Limiting toxin exposure helps support internal and external health.

11. Maintain a Positive Outlook:
- Foster a positive mindset and focus on gratitude. Maintaining a hopeful and optimistic outlook can contribute to emotional resilience and a youthful perspective on life.

12. Regular Health Check-ups:
- Schedule regular health check-ups and screenings. Proactive healthcare and early detection of potential issues contribute to overall well-being.

13. Cultivate Joyful Activities:
- Engage in activities that bring you joy and fulfillment. Whether it's pursuing hobbies, spending time in nature, or connecting with loved ones, cultivating joy contributes to a vibrant and youthful spirit.

14. Posture and Movement:
- Be mindful of your posture and incorporate movements that promote flexibility and balance. Maintaining good posture and staying physically active contribute to a more youthful appearance and overall vitality.

15. Laugh and Have fun:
- Incorporate laughter and moments of joy into your daily life. Laughter is not only good for the soul but also has potential health benefits, including stress reduction and improved mood.

By integrating these lifestyle habits into your daily routine, you can foster youthful vitality that extends beyond physical appearance to encompass holistic well-being. It's essential to tailor these habits to your individual needs and preferences, creating a sustainable and enjoyable approach to a vibrant life.

Stress management

In the hustle and bustle of our modern lives, stress has become an inevitable companion. Balancing work, relationships, and personal well-being can often feel like navigating a complex maze. However, understanding and implementing effective stress management techniques can pave the way for a calmer, more centered existence.

The Impact of Stress
Stress, when left unchecked, can have profound effects on both mental and physical well-being. From sleep disturbances to heightened anxiety, and even more severe health issues, chronic stress can take a toll on various aspects of our lives. Recognizing the signs and acknowledging the importance of managing stress is the first step toward creating a healthier and more resilient self.

Mindfulness and Meditation
One powerful avenue for stress management is the practice of mindfulness and meditation. These techniques encourage individuals to stay present in the moment, fostering a deep connection with one's thoughts and feelings. Mindfulness, often achieved through practices like deep breathing or guided meditation, can help break the cycle of anxious thoughts and promote a sense of calm.

Physical Activity as a Stress Reliever
Regular physical activity is not only beneficial for physical health but also plays a crucial role in stress management. Exercise releases endorphins, the body's natural mood elevators, and provides an outlet for pent-up tension. Whether it's a brisk walk, a yoga session, or a full-body workout, incorporating movement into daily life can significantly reduce stress levels.

The Power of a Support System
Social connections are fundamental to our well-being, and they can be a potent antidote to stress. Sharing thoughts and concerns with friends, family, or a therapist provides an emotional outlet. A supportive network can offer perspectives, advice, or simply a listening ear, fostering a sense of community and understanding.

Time Management and Prioritization
Feeling overwhelmed is a common trigger for stress. Developing effective time management skills and prioritizing tasks can help create a sense of control. Breaking down larger tasks into smaller, manageable steps and setting realistic goals contribute to a more structured and less stressful daily routine.

Relaxation Techniques
Incorporating relaxation techniques into daily life can significantly impact stress levels. Techniques such as progressive muscle relaxation, visualization, or even taking a few moments for deep breathing can induce a state of calmness. These practices serve as quick respites in the midst of a hectic day.

Nourishing the Body with Healthy Habits
A well-nourished body is better equipped to handle stress. Consuming a balanced diet, staying hydrated, and minimizing the intake of stimulants like caffeine and sugar can contribute to physical resilience. Additionally, ensuring adequate sleep is essential, as quality rest plays a pivotal role in stress recovery.

Setting Boundaries
Learning to say 'no' and setting healthy boundaries is a key aspect of stress management. Overcommitting to responsibilities can lead to burnout and increased stress levels. Understanding personal limits and communicating them effectively helps create a more sustainable and balanced lifestyle.

Seeking Professional Guidance
When stress becomes overwhelming or chronic, seeking professional guidance is a proactive step toward effective management. Mental health professionals, such as psychologists or counselors, can provide valuable tools and strategies tailored to individual needs.

Conclusion
Stress management emerges as a crucial thread, weaving together the various elements that contribute to our well-being. By incorporating mindfulness, maintaining social connections, and adopting healthy habits, individuals can cultivate resilience in the face of life's challenges. Stress, rather than an insurmountable adversary, becomes an opportunity for growth and self-discovery, ultimately leading to a more harmonious and fulfilling life.

Quality sleep rejuvenation

Quality sleep is not just a period of rest; it's a vital cornerstone of overall well-being and rejuvenation. Achieving restorative sleep involves more than just clocking in hours; it encompasses various factors that contribute to physical, mental, and emotional revitalization.

Understanding Quality Sleep
Quality sleep goes beyond the duration; it's about the depth and effectiveness of each sleep cycle. During a good night's sleep, the body undergoes essential processes such as tissue repair, hormone regulation, and memory consolidation. Here are key aspects to consider for achieving quality sleep rejuvenation:

1. Consistent Sleep Schedule:
Maintain a consistent sleep schedule by going to bed and waking up at the same time every day, even on weekends. This helps regulate the body's internal clock, promoting a more stable sleep-wake cycle.

2. Creating a Restful Environment:
Design your sleep environment to be conducive to rest. Keep the bedroom cool, dark, and quiet.
Invest in a comfortable mattress and pillows to support proper sleep posture.
3. Limiting Stimulants and Electronics:
Reduce or eliminate stimulants like caffeine and nicotine, especially in the hours leading up to
bedtime. Additionally, minimize screen time before sleep, as the blue light emitted from
electronic devices can interfere with melatonin production, a hormone crucial for sleep.
4. Establishing a Pre-Sleep Routine:
Develop a calming pre-sleep routine to signal to your body that it's time to wind down. This
could include activities such as reading a book, taking a warm bath, or practicing relaxation
techniques.
5. Balanced Diet:
Maintain a balanced diet, and avoid heavy meals close to bedtime. Certain foods, like those rich
in tryptophan (found in turkey, nuts, and seeds), can promote relaxation and aid in quality sleep.
6. Regular Exercise:
Engage in regular physical activity, but try to complete vigorous exercise earlier in the day.
Exercise can promote better sleep, but intense workouts too close to bedtime may have the
opposite effect.
7. Mindfulness and Stress Reduction:
Incorporate mindfulness or relaxation techniques into your evening routine. Practices such as
deep breathing, meditation, or gentle yoga can help calm the mind and reduce stress,
contributing to a more rejuvenating sleep experience.
8. Limiting Naps:
If you nap during the day, keep it short (around 20-30 minutes) and earlier in the day to avoid
interfering with nighttime sleep. Napping can be beneficial, but excessive or late-day napping
may disrupt your sleep cycle.
9. Understanding Sleep Cycles:
Sleep occurs in cycles, including REM (Rapid Eye Movement) and non-REM stages. Aim for a
balance of both to experience the full benefits of sleep. These cycles are crucial for memory
consolidation, learning, and overall rejuvenation.
10. Seeking Professional Guidance:
- If persistent sleep issues arise, consider seeking professional guidance. Sleep disorders or
chronic insomnia may require evaluation and intervention from a healthcare professional.
Quality sleep rejuvenation is a multifaceted endeavor that involves cultivating healthy sleep
habits and prioritizing the factors that contribute to a restful night.

Continuing the journey of youthful living

Continuing the journey of youthful living is a commitment to ongoing self-care, holistic well-being, and a mindset that embraces the full spectrum of life's experiences. As we navigate the intricacies of maintaining vitality, several key principles can guide us on this enriching path.

1. Lifelong Learning:
Embrace a spirit of curiosity and continuous learning. Whether exploring new interests, acquiring skills, or staying abreast of current developments, a curious mind keeps us engaged and adaptable.
2. Cultivating Resilience:
Life is filled with challenges, and cultivating resilience is fundamental to youthful living. Approach setbacks as opportunities for growth, learn from experiences, and develop a positive mindset that fosters adaptability.
3. Mindful Nutrition:
Maintain a mindful approach to nutrition. Focus on nourishing your body with a variety of nutrient-rich foods, paying attention to how your choices impact your overall health and energy levels.
4. Hybrid Fitness:
Evolve your fitness routine to suit your changing needs. Incorporate a mix of cardiovascular exercises, strength training, and flexibility routines. Listen to your body and adapt your workouts to promote lifelong physical well-being.
5. Holistic Health Check-ups:
Regular health check-ups are not just for detecting issues but for proactive wellness. Schedule routine visits to healthcare professionals, focusing not only on physical health but also mental and emotional well-being.
6. Connection and Community:
Foster meaningful connections with others. Engage in community activities, nurture friendships, and share experiences. Social connections contribute significantly to emotional well-being and a sense of purpose.
7. Mind-Body Practices:
Explore mind-body practices like yoga, meditation, or tai chi. These practices not only promote physical health but also cultivate mindfulness, reduce stress, and contribute to a sense of balance.
8. Embracing Change:
Youthful living involves embracing change with open arms. Recognize that life is dynamic, and adapting to new circumstances, challenges, and opportunities is a vital aspect of staying youthful.
9. Joyful Pursuits:
Continue to engage in activities that bring you joy. Whether it's pursuing hobbies, traveling, or exploring creative outlets, incorporating joy into your life enhances overall happiness and fulfillment.
10. Caring for Mental Health:

- Prioritize mental health by managing stress, seeking support when needed, and fostering a positive mindset. A resilient and positive mental outlook is a cornerstone of youthful living.
11. Mindful Aging:
- Embrace the aging process mindfully. Acknowledge and celebrate the wisdom that comes with age, and let go of societal pressures or unrealistic expectations. Aging is a natural part of life's journey.
12. Gratitude Practice:
- Cultivate a gratitude practice. Regularly expressing gratitude for the positive aspects of life fosters a sense of contentment and reinforces a positive outlook.
13. Sustainable Self-Care:
- Prioritize sustainable self-care practices. This involves balancing moments of indulgence with consistent habits that support your physical, mental, and emotional health over the long term.
14. Environmental Consciousness:
- Extend your youthful living ethos to environmental consciousness. Make choices that contribute to a sustainable and eco-friendly lifestyle, promoting not only personal well-being but the health of the planet.
15. Adventurous Spirit:
- Maintain an adventurous spirit. Whether it's trying new activities, exploring new places, or embracing new perspectives, an adventurous approach keeps life dynamic and invigorating.

Continuing the journey of youthful living is an ongoing commitment to self-discovery, growth, and embracing the full richness of life. By integrating these principles into your lifestyle, you not only nurture your own well-being but also contribute positively to the world around you. It's a journey that evolves with each step, fostering a sense of vibrancy, purpose, and fulfillment throughout the various chapters of life.